RENAL DIET COOKBOOK

A complete guide to renal health

Melissa Monroe

Copyright © 2024 Melissa Monroe

Table of Contents

Introduction to Renal Diet:

Welcome to the world of renal cookery, a gourmet trip that not only tantalizes your taste buds but also nourishes your kidneys! Let's dive into the bright palette of flavors created to celebrate your health and raise your kidney well-being in this introduction.

A renal diet is more than simply a list of "do's" and "don'ts"; it's a symphony of components working together to produce a delicious, kidney-friendly tune. So, what's the inside scoop on this culinary masterpiece?

Consider your kidneys to be unsung heroes working ceaselessly backstage in your body's vast theater. These critical organs play an important role in waste removal, electrolyte balance, and fluid balance. Consider the renal diet to be the director's script, carefully constructed to guarantee the kidneys receive the standing ovation they deserve.

Our gastronomic trip begins with a focus on salt, potassium, and phosphorus management. But don't worry! We're not here to give up flavor for the sake of health. Instead, we're about to embark on a delectable adventure in which every ingredient plays a specific role that has been meticulously organized to keep your kidneys humming a happy tune.

As we turn the pages of this cookbook, we'll find recipes that go beyond the usual, demonstrating that a renal diet can be both fulfilling and delicious. Each recipe is a celebration of balance and taste, from zesty morning pleasures to delicious evening indulgences and even a few guilt-free sweets.

So, dear reader, buckle up and prepare to enter a realm where nutrition meets culinary artistry. Let's relish the delicacies of a renal-friendly lifestyle, making each meal not only a feast for the senses but also a toast to the health of your kidneys' unsung heroes! Cheers to more tasty, kidney-loving adventures!

what is a renal diet?

Consider your kidneys, the extraordinary bean-shaped organs that serve as the unsung heroes of your body's filtration system. They work ceaselessly behind the scenes to remove waste, extra fluids, and electrolytes from the body's blood. Now comes the main character of our story: the renal diet.

A renal diet is a customized menu for your culinary selections that is specifically developed to support good kidney function. It's not just about what you eat; it's about fueling your kidneys with the appropriate substances while keeping sodium, potassium, and phosphorus in check.

Why is it so important, you may ask? Your kidneys crave harmony, and a renal diet is the maestro's wand that creates it. By controlling our nutritional intake, we ensure that our kidneys do not have to work overtime, minimizing extra stress and difficulties.

In layman's words, a renal diet is your VIP ticket to a kidney-friendly lifestyle. It's a proactive way to help these hardworking organs stay in peak shape for the long term. So, as we embark on this culinary journey together, keep in mind that a renal diet is more than simply a collection of rules; it's a delectable dedication to kidney health. Begin the feast for your kidneys!

Managing Sodium and Phosphorus intake

Let's now delve into the renal diet's backstage secrets—the main concepts that set the stage for a kidney-friendly culinary symphony. Consider these principles to be the guiding lights that ensure your kidneys' delicate dance doesn't lose a beat.

1. Sorcery with Sodium:

The naughty magician of water retention, sodium, is a key participant in the renal drama. It is critical to control its intake in order to maintain a good fluid balance. Prepare to become a sodium sorcerer, enchanting your dishes with herbs and spices rather than the salty wand.

2. Potassium Abilities:

Enter potassium, the nutritional superstar who can play both the hero and the villain roles. Potassium balance is critical since too much might affect your heart rhythm. Fear not, daring chef! Our recipes will guide you through the maze of potassium-rich meals, allowing you to find the optimal balance.

3. Phosphorus Dexterity:

Phosphorus, the elusive mineral, can be found in a variety of daily foods. Too much might upset your body's delicate equilibrium, affecting bone health and other areas. Our culinary adventure includes phosphorus finesse, which teaches you how to make careful decisions without sacrificing flavor.

Keep these concepts in mind as you begin on this gastronomic adventure—they're the secret sauce to a kidney-friendly feast. You'll master the art of controlling salt, potassium, and phosphorus intake with a dash of creativity and expertise, guaranteeing your kidneys take center stage in a healthy performance. Allow the culinary magic to begin!

Nutritional Information:

Get ready to uncover the nutritional mysteries of each mouthwatering cuisine in our renal diet cookbook!

We believe in transparency, providing you with the knowledge to make informed choices for your kidney health. Here's what you may expect in the nutritional information section:

1. Sodium Spotlight:

Unmask the salt content in each dish. Sodium plays a key function in fluid equilibrium, but too much can lead to difficulties. We'll give you the skinny on how our recipes keep sodium in check, letting you taste the flavors without excess.

2. Potassium Portrait:

Discover the potassium content, the silent hero that can be a bit of a double-edged blade. Our recipes will guide you through the potassium-rich environment, ensuring your potassium intake is well-managed for a healthy heart and kidneys.

3. Phosphorus Presentation:

Peel back the layers to discover the phosphorous content. Phosphorus, frequently subtle in its presence, is demystified in each recipe. We'll teach you how to enjoy a nice lunch without unwittingly tipping the phosphorous scale.

These nutritional insights are your ticket to a thoughtful culinary experience. Armed with this information, you can adapt your meals to fit your kidney health needs. So, while you read through the pages of our cookbook, consider it your nutritional compass, directing you towards delectable, kidney-friendly selections. Let the feast for your taste buds and kidneys continue!

Portion Control

Yes, let's get into the nitty gritty of portion control, ensuring that each serving size is designed to meet your kidney health goals.

1. Plate Precision:

Our cookbook's serving sizes are precisely calculated. There are precise measurements for each ingredient, leaving no opportunity for error. This precision is your ally in keeping a balanced diet without sacrificing taste.

2. Proportional Balance:

We believe in the power of balance. Each recipe proposes serving amounts that maintain a balanced distribution of macronutrients—proteins, carbs, and fats. This balance is intended to keep your kidneys happy and your taste buds happy.

3. Visual Cues:

Not a fan of measuring cups? No need to be concerned! Our cookbook includes visual hints to help you estimate portion proportions with a fast scan. These clues, whether the size of a deck of cards for proteins or the circumference of a tennis ball for fruits, make portion control a simple.

4. Customizable Options:

We recognize that one size does not fit all. Our recipes are adaptable, allowing you to change serving amounts based on your specific needs. We have a hearty lunch or a lighter alternative for you.

5. Mindful Eating Strategies:

In addition to portion numbers, our cookbook provides mindful eating recommendations. Take your time, taste each bite, and pay attention to your body's instincts. Portion control is more than just counting calories; it's about developing a thoughtful relationship with food.

6. Nutritional Information Per Serving:

We provide nutritional facts per serving to better empower you. This contains not only the total sodium, potassium, and phosphorus content, but also the breakdown of calories and other vital nutrients. Knowledge is your most powerful ally in making educated decisions.

Consider our cookbook a valued partner on your quest to portion management mastery, rather than merely a recipe reference. Allow exact measurements, visual clues, and flexible options to be your allies in producing kidney-friendly meals that are as enjoyable for your health as they are for your taste buds. Happy and careful dining!

Ingredient Substitutions:

It's true that being adaptable is key when it comes to modifying meals for a renal diet. With a helpful guidance on ingredient replacements in our cookbook, we've got you covered so your culinary creations stay delicious without sacrificing kidney health. Here are a few crucial substitutions:

1. Power Plays with Potassium:

- Replace bananas with berries or apples to add some sweetness.
- Sweet potatoes or cauliflower are lower in potassium than regular potatoes.
- Try red bell peppers with tomatoes for a taste and color explosion.

2. Twists Appropriate for Phosphorus:

- Dairy: Use non-dairy substitutes, such as rice or almond milk.
- Nuts and Seeds: Go for lower-phosphorus choices like pine nuts or sunflower seeds.
- Whole Grains: Consider grains such as bulgur or quinoa rather than those with greater phosphorus content.

3. Deceptive Sodium Fixations:

- Use tamari or low-sodium soy sauce instead of regular soy sauce.
- Canned Beans: To reduce salt intake, use dried beans that you prepare yourself.

- Processed Meats: Steer clear of cured or processed meats in favor of fresh, lean cuts.

4. Marvels of Herbs and Spices:
- Salt: Spices like cumin or turmeric, together with herbs like thyme and rosemary, can enhance flavor.
- Seasoning Mixtures: Make your own mixes using onion and garlic powders as well as other low-sodium herbs.

5. Secret Treasures in Grains:
- Brown Rice: Try it with white rice or other grains, such as barley or couscous.
- Look into substitutes for whole wheat flour, such as oat or almond flour.

Recall that the goal of these changes is to broaden your gastronomic horizons rather than to impose restrictions. Use your imagination and use these substitutes' tastes to take your creations to new heights. These substitutions turn your kitchen into a tasty, kidney-friendly artistry!

Meal Planning Tips:

Of course! Let's give those meal planning suggestions a modern makeover:

1. The Balanced Plate Art:

Turn your meal into a canvas where colorful veggies, nutritious grains, and lean proteins interact in a harmonious dance. Aim for balance by making sure that every meal is a masterwork of healthy fats, carbohydrates, and protein.

2. Symphony of Nutrients:

Share the passion of nutrition all day long. Make a daily symphony where potassium, phosphorus, and other essentials take turns being the focus instead of cramming all the nutrients into one meal.

3. Rotating Proteins:

Switching up your protein sources will keep your tastebuds interested. Adding variety to your meals guarantees a varied intake of nutrients and helps you get rid of meal boredom. Think about things like juicy poultry or the adaptable tofu.

4. Ability to Portion:

Learn the secrets of portion control. Choose more frequent, smaller meals to support your kidneys' effective nutrient management and continuous energy flow.

5. The Vegetable Spectrum:

Cover your dish with a rainbow of vegetables. Every hue offers a special nutritional reward. Allow the oranges, greens, and reds to come together to form an eye-catching, nutrient-dense masterpiece.

6. Elegance of Hydration:

Accept hydration as a creative medium. To keep your kidneys happy, drink enough of water throughout the day and eat plenty of hydrating foods like oranges, cucumbers, and melons.

7. Conscientious Eating:

Choose kidney-friendly snacks like yogurt, fresh fruit, and unsalted nuts to elevate munching to a fine art. These munchies provide contentment without taxing your kidneys.

8. Investigating the Kitchen:

Take a gastronomic adventure by trying out some new recipes. Every dinner becomes an interesting culinary experience when you experiment with different cuisines and cooking techniques.

9. Fiber Swelling:

Give fiber, whole grains, fruits, and veggies the spotlight. This contributes a critical element to the entire picture of heart health in addition to helping with digestion.

Variety is the foundation of a dynamic, kidney-conscious diet, not just a flavoring. Accept the diverse range of tastes and nutrients to make every meal a joyous occasion to celebrate your well-being. Cheers to a vibrant, well-rounded, kidney-friendly gastronomic adventure!

Cooking Techniques:

Of course, let's get started with some cooking methods designed for a renal diet cookbook. Two excellent ways to lower the potassium and phosphorus content of some foods are leaching and soaking. Here's a quick rundown:

Leaching: To lower the potassium level of high-potassium foods including potatoes, sweet potatoes, and pumpkin, this method entails soaking them in water. Slice the vegetables into little pieces and let them soak for a few hours in a lot of water. To further lower potassium levels throughout the soaking phase, you can also change the water several times.

Soaking is an excellent method for lowering phosphorus levels in grains, beans, and legumes. Before cooking, give them a good rinse and let them soak in water for a long time. When cooking, discard the soaking water and use fresh water. This aids in phosphorus leaching out.

Boiling: Boiling reduces the amounts of potassium and phosphorus in a variety of foods. After boiling grains and vegetables in lots of water, drain and discard the water. This is particularly useful for rice, as it may be boiled and soaked to reduce its phosphorus content.

Blanching is the process of rapidly cooking vegetables and then submerging them in freezing water. This process lowers the potassium and phosphorus content while preserving part of the texture and color.

Peeling and Chopping: Peeling and chopping produce will also lower potassium levels in the body. For instance, you can make fruits like pears and apples more kidney-friendly by peeling and removing their seeds.

Selecting Low-Phosphorus Ingredients: Whenever feasible, choose low-phosphorus substitutes. For instance, utilize processed grains rather than whole grains and opt for white rice rather than brown rice. Limiting your intake of phosphorus can also be achieved by choosing fresh, lean meats and poultry.

Don't forget to speak with a qualified dietitian or healthcare provider to develop a customized renal diet plan that satisfies unique nutritional requirements.

Easy to follow recipes

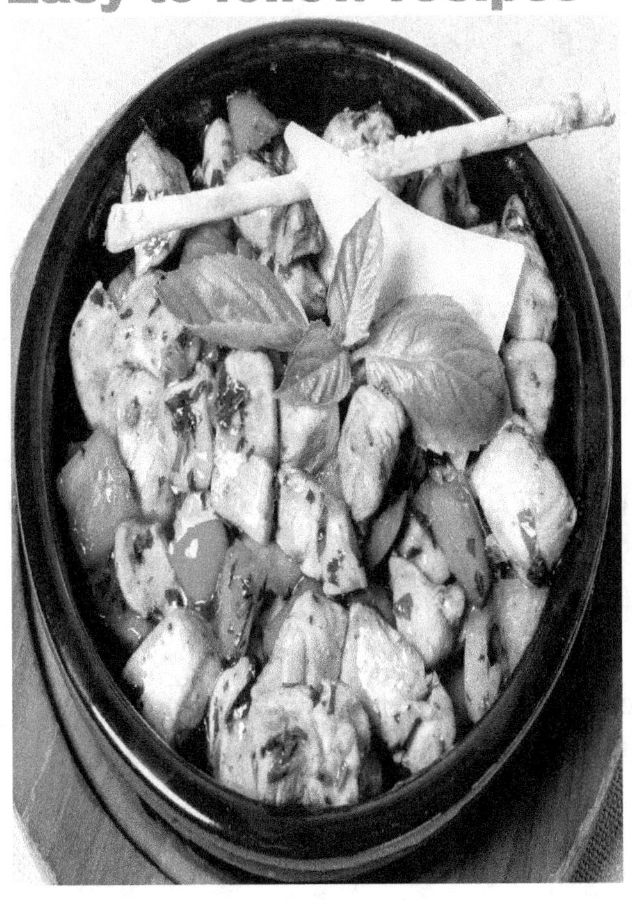

Grilled Chicken Salad with Lemon-Tahini Dressing:

The following is the procedure for preparing Grilled Chicken Salad with Lemon-Tahini Dressing:

Ingredients:

2 chicken breasts without bones or skin

- Four cups of assorted salad greens
- Ingredients: - 1 cup of cherry tomatoes, cut in half - 1 cucumber, sliced - 1/4 cup of thinly sliced red onion - 1/4 cup of crumbled feta cheese (optional)

To make the Lemon-Tahini Dressing:

- 3 tablespoons of tahini
- 2 teaspoons of freshly squeezed lemon juice
- 2 teaspoons water 1 tablespoon olive oil
- 1 minced clove of garlic
- Salt and pepper to taste

Instructions:

- ➢ Preheat the grill to medium-high heat.

- Season the chicken breasts with salt and pepper. Grill for 6-8 minutes per side or until well done. Allow the chicken to rest for a few minutes before slicing it into thin pieces.

- In a large bowl, combine the salad greens, cherry tomatoes, cucumber, and red onion.

- In a small bowl, mix together the tahini, lemon juice, water, olive oil, minced garlic, salt, and pepper until smooth. Adjust the consistency with more water as needed.

- Pour the Lemon-Tahini Dressing over the salad and toss gently to coat the vegetables.

- Arrange the sliced grilled chicken on top of the salad. Sprinkle with crumbled feta cheese if preferred.

- Serve immediately and enjoy your kidney-friendly Grilled Chicken Salad with Lemon-Tahini Dressing!

Quinoa and Vegetable Stir-Fry

Ingredients:

- 1 cup quinoa, rinsed and drained
- 2 cups water or low-sodium vegetable broth 1 tablespoon vegetable oil
- 1 onion, thinly sliced 2 bell peppers (any color), thinly sliced
- 1 zucchini, diced
- 1 cup broccoli florets
- 2 carrots, julienned 3 cloves garlic, minced
- 1/4 cup low-sodium soy sauce
- 1 tablespoon sesame oil
- 1 teaspoon fresh ginger, grated 2 green onions, chopped (for garnish)
- Sesame seeds (optional, for garnish)

Instructions:

➢ In a medium saucepan, add quinoa and water or vegetable broth. Bring to a boil, then decrease heat to low, cover, and simmer for 15-20 minutes or until quinoa is cooked and water is absorbed. Fluff with a fork and set aside.

➢ In a large wok or skillet, heat vegetable oil over medium-high heat.

➢ Add sliced onions and stir-fry for 2-3 minutes until softened.

➢ Add bell peppers, zucchini, broccoli, and carrots to the wok. Stir-fry for an additional 5-7 minutes or until the vegetables are tender-crisp.

➢ Add minced garlic, grated ginger, soy sauce, and sesame oil to the vegetables. Stir well to mix.

➢ Add the cooked quinoa to the wok and toss everything together until well incorporated and heated through.

➢ Garnish with chopped green onions and sesame seeds, if preferred.

➤ Serve hot and enjoy your kidney-friendly Quinoa and Vegetable Stir-Fry!

Baked Salmon with Dill and Lemon

Ingredients:

- 4 salmon fillets
- 2 tablespoons olive oil
- 2 teaspoons fresh lemon juice
- 2 cloves garlic, minced
- 1 tablespoon fresh dill, chopped
- Salt and pepper to taste
- Lemon slices (for garnish)

Instructions:

➤ Preheat the oven to 375°F (190°C). Line a baking sheet with parchment paper.

➤ Place the salmon fillets on the prepared baking sheet.

➢ In a small bowl, whisk together olive oil, lemon juice, minced garlic, chopped dill, salt, and pepper.

➢ Brush the salmon fillets with the lemon-dill mixture, ensuring they are uniformly coated.

➢ Place a lemon slice on top of each salmon fillet for added taste.

➢ Bake in the preheated oven for 12-15 minutes or until the salmon flakes easily with a fork.

➢ Optional: Broil for an extra 2-3 minutes for a golden crust on top.

➢ Remove from the oven and let it rest for a few minutes before serving.

➢ Garnish with additional fresh dill and lemon slices if preferred.

> Serve your kidney-friendly Baked Salmon with Dill and Lemon alongside your favorite low-phosphorus side dishes. Enjoy!

Egg White Omelette with Spinach and Tomatoes

Ingredients:

- 4 egg whites
- 1 cup fresh spinach, chopped
- 1/2 cup cherry tomatoes, halved
- 1/4 cup onion, finely chopped
- 1/4 cup bell pepper, finely chopped
- 1 tablespoon olive oil
- Salt and pepper to taste
- Fresh herbs (such as parsley or chives) for garnish

Instructions:

- ➢ In a bowl, whisk the egg whites until foamy. Season with salt and pepper.

- ➢ Heat olive oil in a non-stick skillet over medium heat.

- ➢ Add chopped onion and bell pepper to the skillet and sauté until softened.

- ➢ Add chopped spinach and cherry tomatoes to the skillet. Cook for an additional 2-3 minutes until the spinach wilts and the tomatoes soften.

- ➢ Pour the whisked egg whites over the vegetables in the skillet.

- ➢ Allow the eggs to set slightly around the edges. Gently raise the edges with a spatula, letting the uncooked egg run below.

- ➢ Once the omelette is mostly set, fold it in half with the spatula.

- ➢ Cook for another minute or until the egg whites are entirely set but still wet.

- ➢ Slide the omelette onto a platter and decorate with fresh herbs.

> ➢ Serve your kidney-friendly Egg White Omelette with Spinach and Tomatoes hot and have a delicious, low-phosphorus meal!

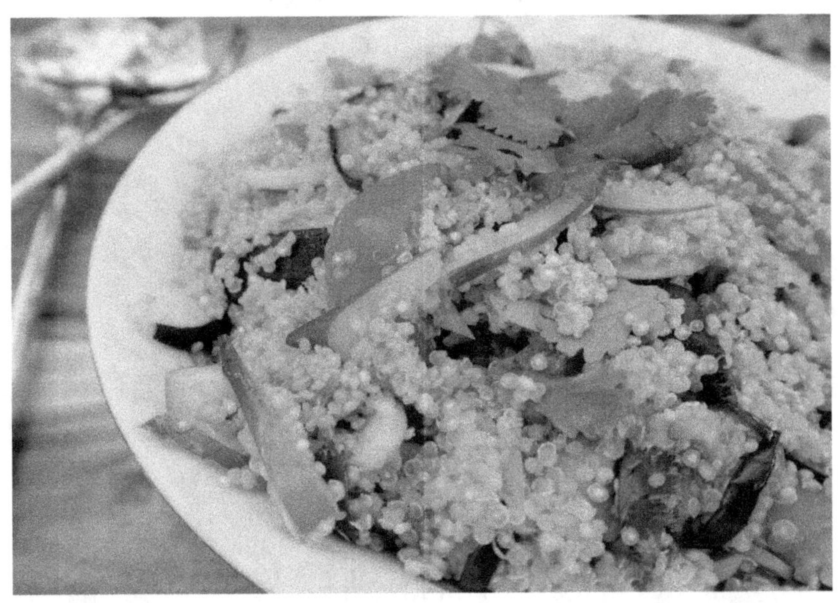

Turkey and Vegetable Skewers

Ingredients:

- 1 pound lean turkey breast, cut into cubes
- 1 zucchini, sliced
- 1 red bell pepper, cut into pieces
- 1 yellow bell pepper, cut into pieces
- 1 red onion, cut into wedges
- 2 tablespoons olive oil
- 2 tablespoons balsamic vinegar
- 1 teaspoon dried oregano
- 1 teaspoon garlic powder
- Salt and pepper to taste
- Wooden or metal skewers

Instructions:

- If using wooden skewers, soak them in water for at least 30 minutes to prevent scorching.

- Preheat your grill or grill pan over medium-high heat.

➢ In a bowl, mix olive oil, balsamic vinegar, dried oregano, garlic powder, salt, and pepper to prepare the marinade.

➢ Thread the turkey cubes, zucchini slices, bell pepper pieces, and red onion wedges onto the skewers, alternating for a colorful presentation.

➢ Brush the skewers with the marinade, ensuring they are well coated.

➢ Grill the skewers for about 10-12 minutes, rotating periodically, or until the turkey is cooked through and the veggies are soft.

➢ Remove from the grill and let them rest for a few minutes.

➢ Serve your kidney-friendly Turkey and Vegetable Skewers with a serving of your favorite low-phosphorus grains or a fresh salad.

Enjoy this tasty and protein-packed dinner!

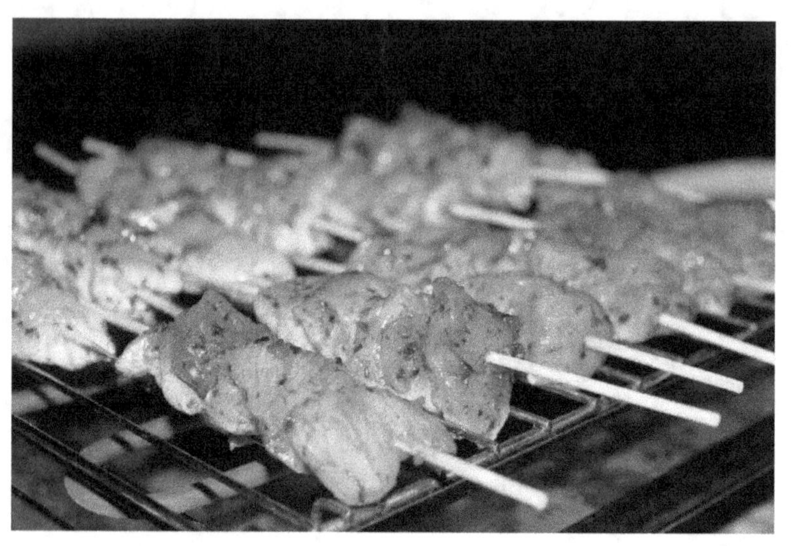

Lentil Soup with Carrots and Celery

Ingredients:

- 1 cup dried green or brown lentils, rinsed and drained
- 1 onion, finely chopped
- 2 carrots, diced 2 celery stalks, diced 3 cloves garlic, minced
- 6 cups low-sodium vegetable broth
- 1 can (14 oz) diced tomatoes, undrained
- 1 teaspoon ground cumin
- 1 teaspoon dried thyme
- 1/2 teaspoon smoked paprika
- Salt and pepper to taste
- 2 tablespoons olive oil
- Fresh parsley for garnish (optional)

Instructions:

- ➢ In a big pot, heat olive oil over medium heat. Add chopped onions, carrots, and celery. Sauté for 5-7 minutes until the vegetables are softened.

- Add minced garlic and sauté for an additional minute until fragrant.

- Stir in lentils, vegetable broth, diced tomatoes, cumin, thyme, smoked paprika, salt, and pepper.

- Bring the soup to a boil, then decrease the heat to low, cover, and simmer for 25-30 minutes or until the lentils are cooked.

- Taste and adjust the seasoning if necessary.

- If you like a smoother texture, you can use an immersion blender to partially puree the soup, leaving some lentils and veggies whole.

- Ladle the kidney-friendly Lentil Soup into dishes, top with fresh parsley if preferred, and serve hot.

- Enjoy a delicious and nutritious cup of soup that's mild on the kidneys!

Roasted Vegetable and Chickpea Bowl

Ingredients:

- 1 can (15 oz) chickpeas, drained and rinsed
- 1 sweet potato, peeled and cubed 1 red bell pepper, cut 1 zucchini, sliced 1 red onion, thinly sliced
- 3 tablespoons olive oil
- 1 teaspoon ground cumin
- 1 teaspoon smoked paprika
- Salt and pepper to taste
- 2 cups cooked quinoa or brown rice
- Fresh lemon slices for serving

Instructions:

➢ Preheat the oven to 400°F (200°C).

➢ In a large mixing basin, combine chickpeas, sweet potato cubes, chopped red bell pepper, zucchini, and red onion.

- Drizzle olive oil over the vegetables and chickpeas. Sprinkle with ground cumin, smoked paprika, salt, and pepper. Toss until everything is well covered.

- Spread the mixture evenly on a baking sheet lined with parchment paper.

- Roast in the preheated oven for 25-30 minutes or until the veggies are soft and chickpeas are golden brown, tossing halfway through.

- While the vegetables are roasting, make quinoa or brown rice according to package instructions.

- Divide the cooked quinoa or brown rice among serving bowls.

- Top with the roasted veggie and chickpea mixture.

- Squeeze fresh lemon juice over the bowl before serving for a burst of citrus flavor.

> Enjoy your kidney-friendly Roasted Vegetable and Chickpea Bowl, full with fiber and nutrients!

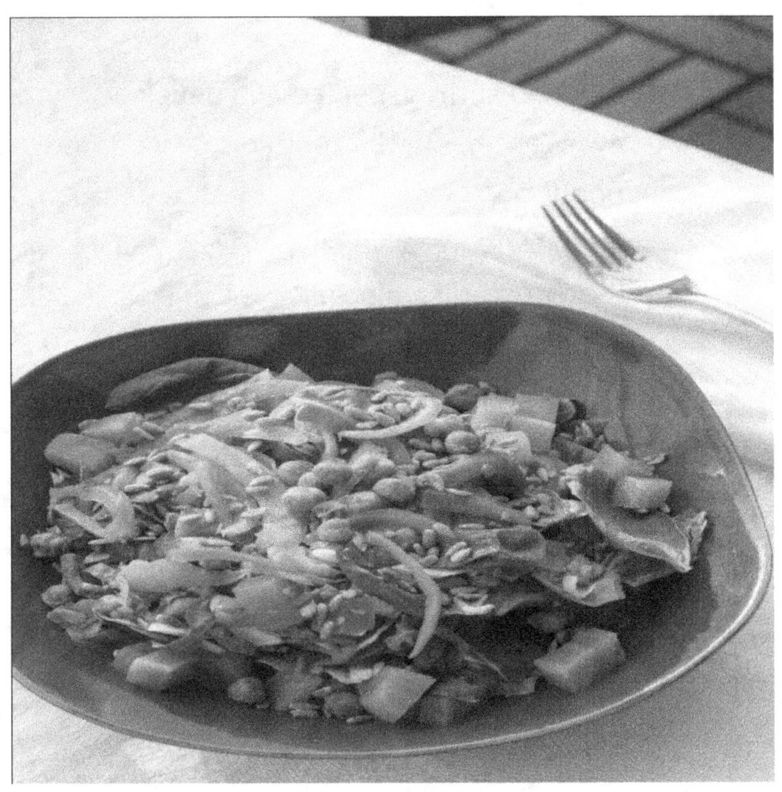

Shrimp and Zucchini Noodles

Ingredients:

- 1 pound shrimp, peeled and deveined
- 4 medium-sized zucchinis, spiralized into noodles
- 2 tablespoons olive oil
- 3 cloves garlic, minced
- 1 teaspoon lemon zest 2 tablespoons fresh lemon juice
- 1/2 teaspoon red pepper flakes (optional)
- Salt and pepper to taste
- Fresh parsley for garnish

Instructions:

- In a large skillet, heat olive oil over medium heat.

- Add minced garlic and sauté for about 1 minute until fragrant.

➢ Add shrimp to the skillet and cook for 2-3 minutes on each side until they turn pink and opaque.

➢ Season the shrimp with lemon zest, lemon juice, red pepper flakes (if using), salt, and pepper. Toss to coat evenly.

➢ Add the zucchini noodles to the skillet and stir with the shrimp and delicious combination. Cook for an additional 2-3 minutes until the zucchini noodles are just soft.

➢ Adjust spice if needed and ensure the noodles are well-coated with the lemony sauce.

➢ Remove from heat and garnish with fresh parsley.

➢ Serve your Shrimp and Zucchini Noodles immediately, and relish the light and aromatic tastes!

Herbed Grilled Tilapia

Ingredients:

- 4 tilapia fillets
- 2 tablespoons olive oil
- 2 teaspoons fresh lemon juice
- 2 cloves garlic, minced
- 1 teaspoon dried oregano
- 1 teaspoon dried thyme
- Salt and pepper to taste
- Lemon wedges for serving
- Fresh parsley for garnish

Instructions:

- In a small bowl, whisk together olive oil, lemon juice, minced garlic, dried oregano, dried thyme, salt, and pepper.

- Place the tilapia fillets in a shallow dish and pour the marinade over them. Ensure each fillet is well-coated. Let them marinade for at least 15-20 minutes.

➢ Preheat your grill or grill pan over medium-high heat.

➢ Grill the tilapia fillets for 3-4 minutes per side or until they readily flake with a fork and have excellent grill marks.

➢ Remove off the grill and transfer to a serving plate.

➢ Garnish with fresh parsley and serve with lemon wedges on the side.

➢ Enjoy your Herbed Grilled Tilapia, a light and delicious alternative for kidney-friendly meals!

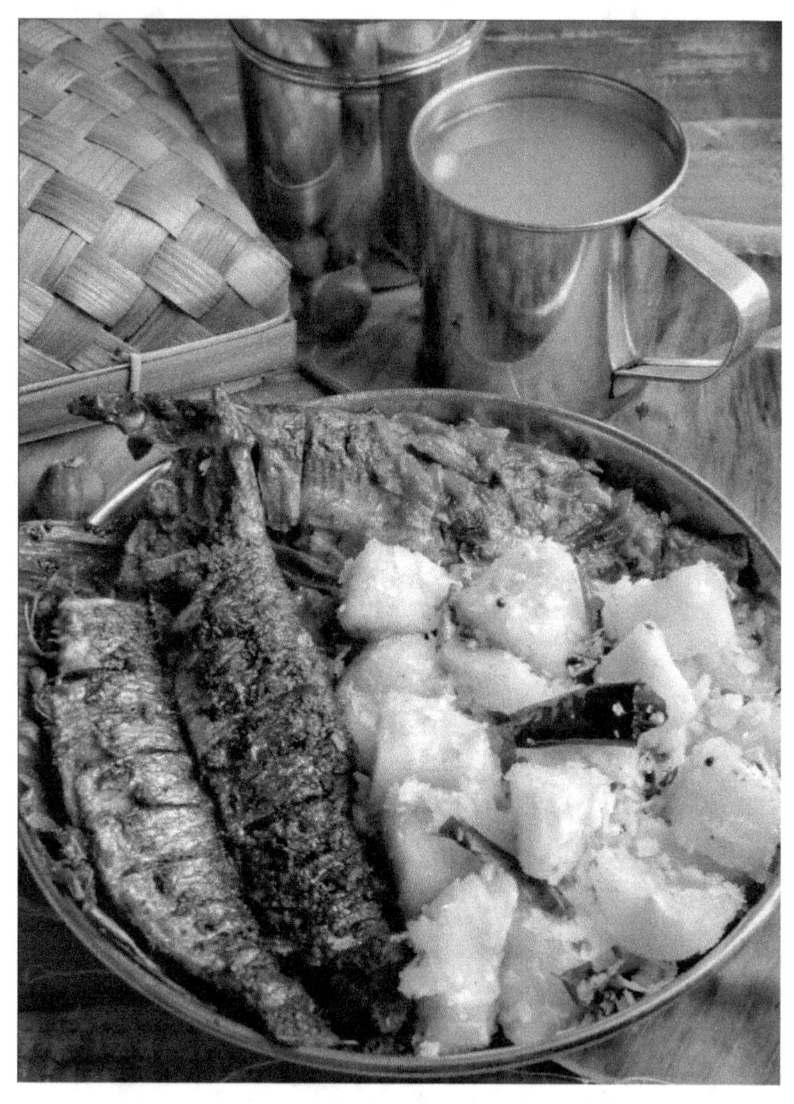

Cauliflower Rice Pilaf

Ingredients:

- 1 medium-sized cauliflower, grated or made into rice
- 1 tablespoon olive oil
- 1 small onion, coarsely chopped
- 2 cloves garlic, minced
- 1/4 cup slivered almonds
- 1/4 cup dried cranberries (unsweetened)
- 1 teaspoon ground cumin
- 1 teaspoon ground coriander
- Salt and pepper to taste
- Fresh parsley for garnish

Instructions:

- Grate or grind the cauliflower into rice-sized pieces.

- In a large skillet, heat olive oil over medium heat.

➢ Add chopped onion and sauté until softened, about 3-4 minutes.

➢ Add minced garlic and slivered almonds to the skillet. Sauté for an additional 2-3 minutes until the almonds are lightly toasted.

➢ Stir in the cauliflower rice, dried cranberries, ground cumin, ground coriander, salt, and pepper.

➢ Cook for 5-7 minutes, stirring periodically, until the cauliflower rice is soft but not mushy.

➢ Adjust spice if needed and sprinkle with fresh parsley.

➢ Serve your kidney-friendly Cauliflower Rice Pilaf as a delightful and nutrient-packed side dish!

Chicken and Vegetable Kebabs

Ingredients:

- 1 pound boneless, skinless chicken breast, cut into chunks
- 1 zucchini, sliced
- 1 red bell pepper, cut into pieces
- 1 yellow bell pepper, cut into pieces
- 1 red onion, cut into wedges
- 2 tablespoons olive oil
- 2 tablespoons balsamic vinegar
- 1 teaspoon dried oregano
- 1 teaspoon garlic powder
- Salt and pepper to taste
- Wooden or metal skewers

Instructions:

- ➢ If using wooden skewers, soak them in water for at least 30 minutes to prevent scorching.

- ➤ In a bowl, whisk together olive oil, balsamic vinegar, dried oregano, garlic powder, salt, and pepper to prepare the marinade.

- ➤ Thread the chicken chunks, zucchini slices, bell pepper chunks, and red onion wedges onto the skewers, alternating for a colorful appearance.

- ➤ Brush the skewers with the marinade, ensuring they are well coated.

- ➤ Preheat your grill or grill pan over medium-high heat.

- ➤ Grill the skewers for about 10-12 minutes, rotating periodically, or until the chicken is cooked through and the vegetables are soft.

- ➤ Remove from the grill and let them rest for a few minutes.

- ➤ Serve your kidney-friendly Chicken and Vegetable Kebabs with a side of brown rice or quinoa for a balanced dinner.

> ➢ Enjoy the amazing flavors of these grilled kebabs!

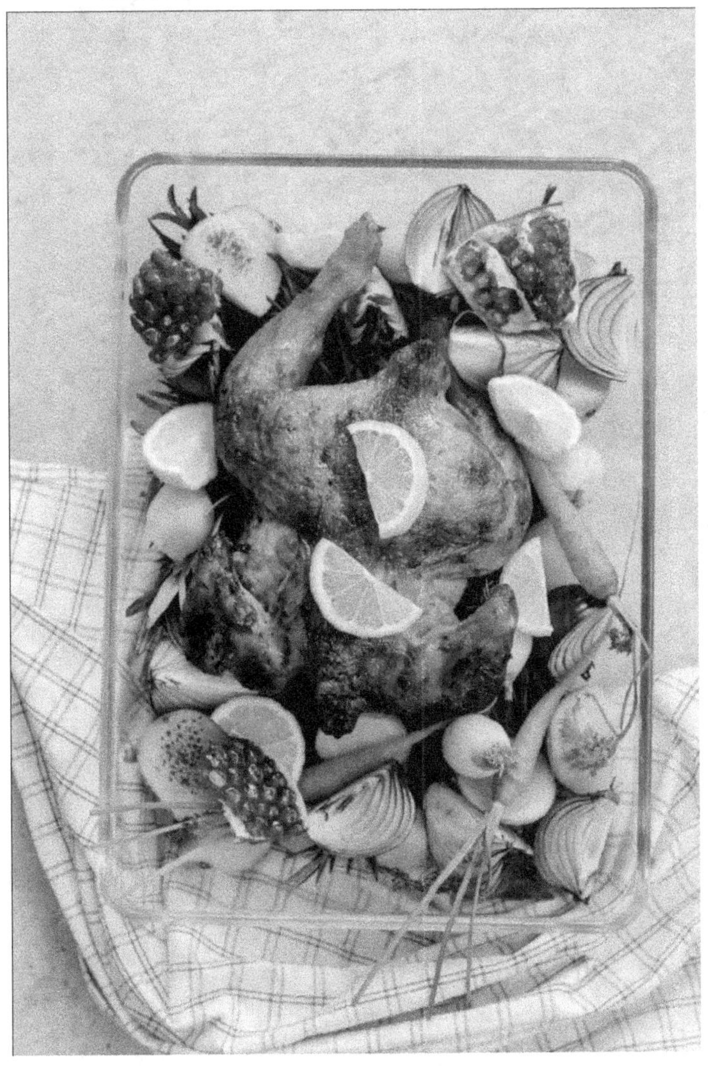

Spinach and Feta Stuffed Chicken Breast

Ingredients:

- 4 boneless, skinless chicken breasts
- 2 cups fresh spinach, chopped
- 1/2 cup crumbled feta cheese
- 2 cloves garlic, minced
- 1 tablespoon olive oil
- 1 teaspoon dried oregano
- Salt and pepper to taste
- Toothpicks or kitchen twine

Instructions:

➢ Preheat the oven to 375°F (190°C).

➢ In a skillet, heat olive oil over medium heat. Add minced garlic and sauté for 1-2 minutes until fragrant.

- ➢ Add chopped spinach to the skillet and simmer until wilted. Remove from heat and let it cool.

- ➢ In a bowl, combine the wilted spinach with crumbled feta, dried oregano, salt, and pepper.

- ➢ Lay the chicken breasts flat and make a horizontal cut down the center, forming a pocket without cutting all the way through.

- ➢ Stuff each chicken breast with the spinach and feta mixture.

- ➢ Secure the aperture with toothpicks or tie with kitchen thread.

- ➢ Season the outside of the chicken breasts with a little of salt and pepper.

- ➢ Heat a skillet over medium-high heat. Brown the filled chicken breasts on each side for 2-3 minutes.

> Transfer the browned chicken breasts to a baking dish and bake in the preheated oven for 20-25 minutes or until the chicken is cooked through.

> Remove toothpicks or twine before serving.

> Serve your Spinach and Feta Stuffed Chicken Breast with a side of steamed veggies or a light salad for a lovely kidney-friendly supper!

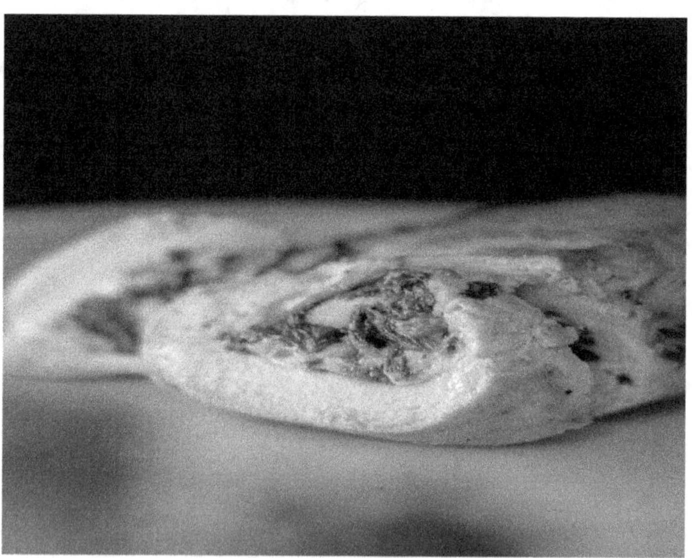

Cucumber and Avocado Salad

Ingredients:

- 2 large cucumbers, peeled and chopped
- 2 ripe avocados, chopped
- 1/4 cup red onion, finely chopped
- 1/4 cup fresh cilantro, chopped 2 tablespoons lime juice
- 2 tablespoons olive oil
- Salt and pepper to taste

Instructions:

- ➤ In a large bowl, add diced cucumbers, diced avocados, chopped red onion, and fresh cilantro.

- ➤ In a small bowl, whisk together lime juice, olive oil, salt, and pepper.

- ➤ Pour the dressing over the cucumber and avocado combination.

➢ Gently toss everything together until well combined.

➢ Taste and adjust the seasoning if needed.

➢ Chill in the refrigerator for about 15-20 minutes to let the flavors mingle.

➢ Serve your kidney-friendly Cucumber and Avocado Salad as a delicious side dish or a light snack.

➢ Enjoy the sharpness of cucumber and the smoothness of avocado in every bite!

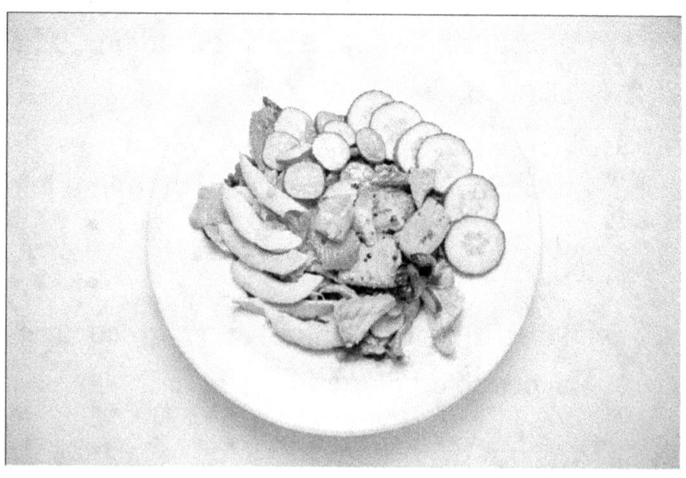

Mediterranean Quinoa Salad

Ingredients:

- 1 cup quinoa, rinsed and drained
- 2 cups water or low-sodium vegetable broth 1 cup cherry tomatoes, halved 1 cucumber, diced 1/2 cup Kalamata olives, sliced 1/4 cup red onion, coarsely chopped
- 1/4 cup feta cheese, crumbled
- 1/4 cup fresh parsley, chopped

For the Dressing:

- 3 tablespoons olive oil
- 2 teaspoons red wine vinegar
- 1 teaspoon dried oregano
- Salt and pepper to taste

Instructions:

➢ In a medium saucepan, add quinoa and water or vegetable broth. Bring to a boil, then decrease heat to low, cover, and simmer for 15-20 minutes or until quinoa is cooked and water is absorbed. Fluff with a fork and let it cool.

➤ In a large bowl, combine chilled quinoa, cherry tomatoes, cucumber, Kalamata olives, red onion, feta cheese, and fresh parsley.

➤ In a small bowl, whisk together olive oil, red wine vinegar, dried oregano, salt, and pepper to create the dressing.

➤ Pour the dressing over the salad and toss lightly to mix.

➤ Adjust the seasoning as needed.

➤ Chill in the refrigerator for at least 30 minutes before serving to enable the flavors to mingle.

➤ Serve your kidney-friendly Mediterranean Quinoa Salad as a light and nutritious main or side dish.

> ➢ Enjoy the colorful colors and Mediterranean-inspired flavors!

Beef and Vegetable Stir-Fry

Ingredients:

- 1 pound lean beef sirloin or flank steak, thinly sliced
- 2 tablespoons soy sauce (low-sodium)
- 1 tablespoon oyster sauce
- 1 tablespoon hoisin sauce
- 1 tablespoon cornstarch
- 2 teaspoons vegetable oil
- 3 cups mixed veggies (broccoli florets, bell peppers, snap peas, carrots), sliced
- 3 cloves garlic, minced
- 1 tablespoon fresh ginger, grated 2 green onions, sliced (for garnish)
- Sesame seeds (optional, for garnish)
- Cooked brown rice or quinoa (for serving)

Instructions:

- ➢ In a bowl, whisk together soy sauce, oyster sauce, hoisin sauce, and cornstarch to form the marinade.

- ➢ Place the sliced beef in the marinade, ensuring each slice is completely coated. Let it marinade for at least 15-20 minutes.

- ➢ Heat 1 tablespoon of vegetable oil in a wok or big skillet over high heat.

- ➢ Add the marinated meat and stir-fry for 2-3 minutes or until browned and cooked through. Remove the steak from the wok and set it aside.

- ➢ In the same skillet, add another tablespoon of vegetable oil.

- ➢ Add minced garlic and grated ginger to the wok, stir-frying for about 1 minute until fragrant.

- Add the mixed veggies to the wok and stir-fry for 4-5 minutes or until they are crisp-tender.

- Return the cooked beef to the wok and stir everything together to incorporate.

- Cook for a another 2 minutes to heat through.

- Garnish with chopped green onions and sesame seeds if preferred.

- Serve your kidney-friendly Beef and Vegetable Stir-Fry over cooked brown rice or quinoa.

- Enjoy the savory and flavorful blend of beef and veggies in this quick and healthful stir-fry!

Lemon Herb Baked Cod

Ingredients:

- 4 cod fillets
- 2 tablespoons olive oil
- 2 teaspoons fresh lemon juice
- 2 cloves garlic, minced
- 1 teaspoon dried thyme
- 1 teaspoon dried rosemary
- Salt and pepper to taste
- Lemon slices (for garnish)
- Fresh parsley (for garnish)

Instructions:

- Preheat the oven to 400°F (200°C).

- Place the cod fillets in a baking dish.

- In a small bowl, whisk together olive oil, fresh lemon juice, minced garlic, dried thyme, dried rosemary, salt, and pepper.

- Pour the lemon herb mixture over the cod fillets, ensuring they are well covered.

➢ Let the fish marinade for about 15 minutes.

➢ Bake in the preheated oven for 15-20 minutes or until the fish is opaque and flakes readily with a fork.

➢ Optional: Broil for an extra 2-3 minutes for a golden crust on top.

➢ Remove from the oven and decorate with lemon slices and fresh parsley.

➢ Serve your kidney-friendly Lemon Herb Baked Cod with a side of steamed veggies or a mild salad.

➢ Enjoy this light and tasty dish that's high in omega-3 fatty acids!

Turkey and Sweet Potato Hash

Ingredients:

- 1 pound ground turkey
- 2 sweet potatoes, peeled and chopped
- 1 onion, finely chopped
- 1 bell pepper, diced
- 2 cloves garlic, minced
- 2 tablespoons olive oil
- 1 teaspoon ground cumin
- 1 teaspoon smoked paprika
- Salt and pepper to taste
- Fresh parsley for garnish

Instructions:

➢ In a large skillet, heat olive oil over medium heat.

➢ Add finely chopped onion and sauté until softened, about 3-4 minutes.

➢ Add ground turkey to the skillet, breaking it up with a spoon. Cook until browned and cooked through.

➢ Stir in minced garlic and simmer for an additional minute until aromatic.

➢ Add diced sweet potatoes and diced bell pepper to the skillet. Cook for 10-12 minutes or until the sweet potatoes are cooked, stirring periodically.

➢ Season the hash with ground cumin, smoked paprika, salt, and pepper. Adjust the seasoning to taste.

➢ Cook for a further 5-7 minutes, allowing the flavors to mingle.

➢ Garnish with fresh parsley before serving.

➢ Serve your kidney-friendly Turkey and Sweet Potato Hash as a wholesome and pleasant supper.

➢ Enjoy the mix of lean turkey, sweet potatoes, and aromatic spices in this delectable hash!

Eggplant Parmesan with Low-Sodium Tomato Sauce

Ingredients:

For the Eggplant Parmesan:

- 2 large eggplants, cut into 1/2-inch rounds
- 2 cups whole wheat breadcrumbs (or almond flour for a lower phosphorus option)
- 1 cup grated Parmesan cheese
- 3 eggs, beaten
- 1 teaspoon dried oregano
- 1 teaspoon dried basil
- Salt and pepper to taste
- Olive oil for baking

For the Low-Sodium Tomato Sauce:

- 2 cups low-sodium tomato sauce
- 2 cloves garlic, minced
- 1 teaspoon dried basil
- 1 teaspoon dried oregano
- Salt and pepper to taste

For Assembly:

- 2 cups mozzarella cheese, shredded

Instructions:

➢ Preheat the oven to 375°F (190°C).

➢ In a small bowl, mix breadcrumbs (or almond flour), grated Parmesan, dried oregano, dried basil, salt, and pepper.

➢ Dip each eggplant slice into the beaten eggs, then coat it in the breadcrumb mixture, pressing lightly to adhere.

➢ Place the oiled eggplant slices on a baking sheet lined with parchment paper.

➢ Drizzle olive oil over the eggplant slices and bake in the preheated oven for 20-25 minutes or until they are golden brown and soft.

➢ While the eggplant is baking, prepare the low-sodium tomato sauce. In a saucepan, add tomato sauce, minced garlic, dried basil, dried oregano, salt, and pepper. Simmer for 10-15 minutes.

- ➤ Once the eggplant is done, remove it from the oven and increase the oven temperature to 400°F (200°C).

- ➤ In a baking dish, put a thin layer of the tomato sauce.

- ➤ Arrange half of the roasted eggplant slices on top of the sauce.

- ➤ Sprinkle half of the shredded mozzarella over the eggplant.

- ➤ Repeat the layers with the remaining eggplant and mozzarella.

- ➤ Bake in the oven for 20-25 minutes or until the cheese is melted and bubbling.

- ➤ Let it cool for a few minutes before serving.

➢ Serve your kidney-friendly Eggplant Parmesan with a side of whole grain pasta or a green salad.

➢ Enjoy this healthier spin on a classic Italian dish!

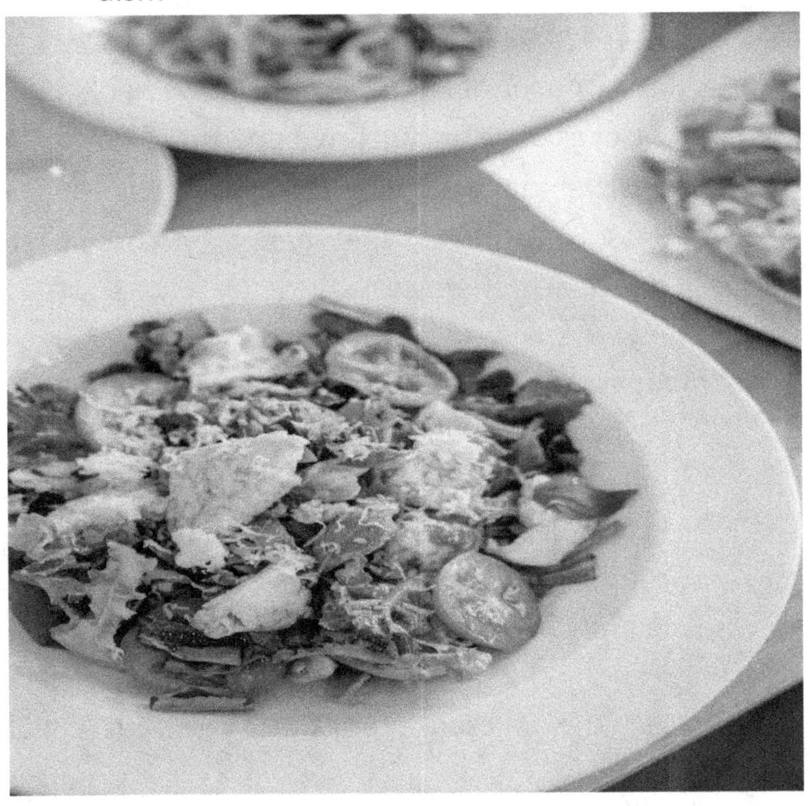

Baked Chicken Drumsticks with Rosemary

Ingredients:

- 8 pieces of chicken drumsticks
- 2 tbsp of olive oil
- 2 teaspoons of freshly chopped rosemary
- 3 cloves of garlic, finely chopped
- 1 tsp lemon zest 1 tbsp lemon juice
- Season with salt and pepper according to personal preference

Instructions:

➢ Preheat the oven to 400°F (200°C).

➢ In a small bowl, combine together olive oil, chopped rosemary, minced garlic, lemon zest, lemon juice, salt, and pepper.

➢ Pat the chicken drumsticks dry with paper towels.

➤ Transfer the drumsticks to a spacious basin and drizzle the rosemary mixture on top of them. Toss until the drumsticks are evenly coated.

➤ Line a baking sheet with parchment paper.

➤ Arrange the drumsticks on the baking sheet in a single layer.

➤ Bake in the preheated oven for 35-40 minutes or until the chicken is golden brown and cooked through, flipping them halfway through.

➤ Check for doneness by putting a meat thermometer into the thickest portion of the drumstick. It should read at least 165°F (74°C).

➤ Remove from the oven and allow the drumsticks rest for a few minutes.

➤ Serve your rosemary-infused Baked Chicken Drumsticks with a side of roasted vegetables or a fresh salad.

➤ Enjoy the aromatic and flavorful tastes of this simple and nutritious dish!

Red Lentil Curry

Ingredients:

- 1 cup red lentils, rinsed and drained
- 1 big onion, coarsely chopped
- 2 tomatoes, chopped 3 cloves garlic, minced
- 1 tablespoon ginger, grated
- 1 can (14 oz) coconut milk
- 1 can (14 oz) diced tomatoes (or use fresh tomatoes)
- 1 tablespoon curry powder
- 1 teaspoon ground cumin
- 1 teaspoon ground coriander
- 1/2 teaspoon turmeric
- 1/2 teaspoon chili powder (adjust to taste)
- 1 tablespoon vegetable oil
- Salt and pepper to taste
- Fresh cilantro for garnish
- Cooked rice or naan for serving

Instructions:

➢ Rinse the red lentils under cold water until the water runs clear. Set aside.

- ➢ In a big pot or Dutch oven, heat vegetable oil over medium heat.

- ➢ Add chopped onions and sauté until they become translucent, about 3-4 minutes.

- ➢ Add minced garlic and grated ginger to the saucepan. Sauté for an additional 1-2 minutes until aromatic.

- ➢ Stir in curry powder, ground cumin, ground coriander, turmeric, and chili powder. Cook for another 1-2 minutes to roast the spices.

- ➢ Add chopped tomatoes to the pot and heat until they start to soften.

- ➢ Pour in the coconut milk and diced tomatoes. Stir well to mix.

- ➢ Add the washed red lentils to the pot. Mix everything together.

➤ Bring the mixture to a boil, then decrease the heat to low, cover, and simmer for about 20-25 minutes or until the lentils are soft and the curry has thickened.

➤ Season with salt and pepper to taste.

➤ Garnish with fresh cilantro before serving.

➤ Serve your Red Lentil Curry over cooked rice or with warm naan.

➤ Enjoy this tasty and healthful curry that's loaded in protein and warming spices!

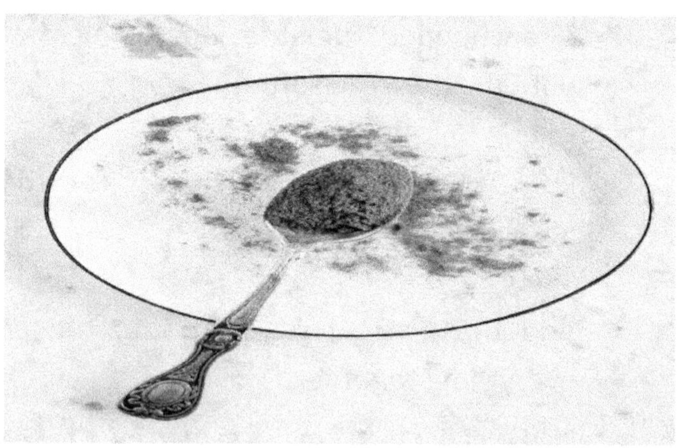

Zucchini and Tomato Frittata

Ingredients:

- 6 big eggs
- 1 zucchini, thinly sliced 1 cup cherry tomatoes, halved 1/2 cup feta cheese, crumbled 1/4 cup fresh basil, chopped 1/4 cup red onion, finely chopped 2 tablespoons olive oil
- Salt and pepper to taste

Instructions:

➢ Preheat your oven to 375°F (190°C).

➢ In a bowl, mix together the eggs. Season with salt and pepper.

➢ Heat olive oil in an oven-safe skillet over medium heat.

➢ Add sliced zucchini to the skillet and cook for 2-3 minutes until slightly mushy.

- Add chopped red onion to the skillet and sauté for an additional 2 minutes.

- Spread the zucchini and onion equally in the skillet.

- Pour the whisked eggs over the zucchini and onion mixture.

- Sprinkle halved cherry tomatoes, crumbled feta, and chopped fresh basil over the eggs.

- Let the frittata cook on the stovetop for 2-3 minutes without stirring.

- Transfer the skillet to the preheated oven and bake for 15-20 minutes or until the frittata is set in the center and slightly browned on top.

- Remove from the oven and let it cool for a few minutes.

- Slice into wedges and serve your Zucchini and Tomato Frittata warm.

- Enjoy a tasty and veggie-packed frittata that makes for a fantastic breakfast or brunch option!

Greek Chicken Souvlaki

Ingredients:

For the Chicken Marinade:

- 1.5 pounds boneless, skinless chicken breasts, cut into cubes
- 1/4 cup olive oil
- 3 tablespoons fresh lemon juice
- 2 tablespoons dried oregano
- 1 teaspoon ground cumin
- 1 teaspoon paprika
- 3 cloves garlic, minced
- Salt and pepper to taste

For the Tzatziki Sauce:

- 1 cup Greek yogurt
- 1 cucumber, grated and squeezed to remove extra moisture
- 2 cloves garlic, minced
- 1 tablespoon fresh dill, chopped 1 tablespoon fresh mint, chopped 1 tablespoon olive oil

- Salt and pepper to taste
-

For Serving:
- Pita bread
- Cherry tomatoes, sliced Red onion, thinly sliced Cucumber, sliced

Instructions:
- ➢ In a bowl, combine olive oil, lemon juice, dried oregano, ground cumin, paprika, minced garlic, salt, and pepper for the chicken marinade.

- ➢ Add the cubed chicken to the marinade, ensuring each piece is well covered. Let it marinade for at least 30 minutes or fridge for a few hours.

- ➢ While the chicken is marinating, prepare the tzatziki sauce. In a bowl, mix Greek yogurt, grated cucumber, minced garlic, chopped dill, chopped mint, olive oil, salt, and pepper. Refrigerate until ready to serve.

➢ Preheat your grill or grill pan over medium-high heat.

➢ Thread the marinated chicken chunks onto skewers.

➢ Grill the chicken skewers for 6-8 minutes, flipping occasionally, until they are cooked through and have a good sear.

➢ Warm the pita bread on the grill for a minute on each side.

➢ Serve the Greek Chicken Souvlaki on warm pita bread, topped with sliced cherry tomatoes, red onion, and cucumber.

➢ Drizzle with the homemade tzatziki sauce.

➢ Enjoy your homemade Greek Chicken Souvlaki with all the fresh and vivid Mediterranean flavors!

Asparagus and Mushroom Stir-Fry

Ingredients:

- 1 bunch asparagus, trimmed and chopped into 2-inch pieces
- 2 cups mushrooms, sliced (button or cremini mushrooms work well)
- 2 tablespoons soy sauce (low-sodium)
- 1 tablespoon hoisin sauce
- 1 tablespoon sesame oil
- 2 cloves garlic, minced
- 1 tablespoon fresh ginger, grated
- 1 tablespoon vegetable oil
- Sesame seeds for garnish (optional)
- Cooked brown rice or quinoa (for serving)

Instructions:

- In a small bowl, mix together soy sauce, hoisin sauce, and sesame oil to produce the sauce.

- Heat vegetable oil in a wok or big skillet over medium-high heat.

➢ Add minced garlic and grated ginger to the wok. Sauté for roughly 1 minute until aromatic.

➢ Add sliced mushrooms to the wok and stir-fry for 2-3 minutes until they begin to soften.

➢ Add asparagus pieces to the wok and continue to stir-fry for an additional 3-4 minutes or until the asparagus is tender-crisp.

➢ Pour the sauce over the vegetables in the wok. Toss everything together to coat evenly.

➢ Cook for an additional 1-2 minutes, allowing the flavors to mingle.

➢ Taste and adjust the seasoning if needed.

➢ Optional: Sprinkle sesame seeds over the stir-fry for extra crunch and taste.

➢ Serve your Asparagus and Mushroom Stir-Fry over cooked brown rice or quinoa.

➢ Enjoy this quick and healthful stir-fry that's packed with nutritious veggies and delicious sauce!

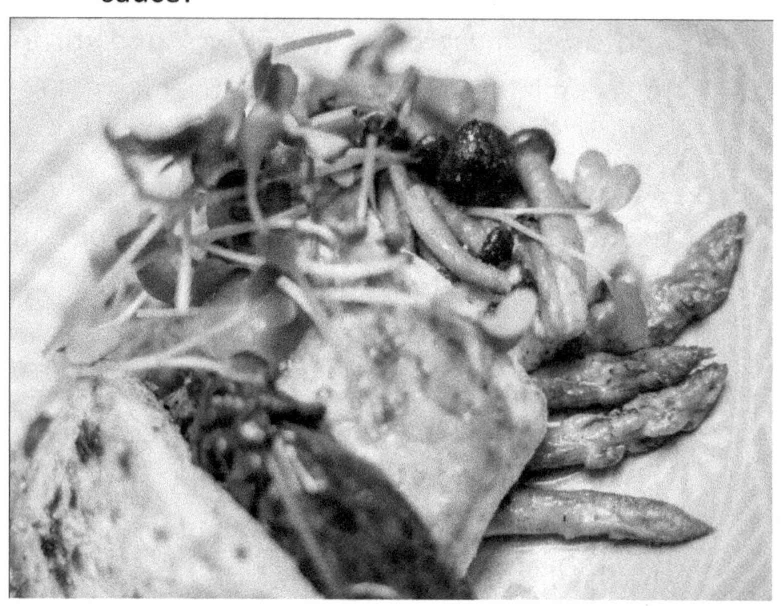

White Bean and Kale Soup

Ingredients:

- 1 tablespoon olive oil
- 1 onion, chopped
- 2 carrots, chopped
- 3 cloves garlic, minced 2 cans (15 oz each) white beans, drained and rinsed (such as cannellini beans)
- 4 cups vegetable broth (low-sodium)
- 1 can (14 oz) chopped tomatoes
- 1 teaspoon dried thyme
- 1 teaspoon dried rosemary
- 1 bay leaf
- Salt and pepper to taste
- 4 cups kale, stems removed and leaves cut
- Fresh lemon juice (optional)
- Grated Parmesan cheese for garnish (optional)

Instructions:

➢ In a big pot, heat olive oil over medium heat.

➤ Add chopped onion and diced carrots to the saucepan. Sauté for 5-7 minutes until the vegetables are softened.

➤ Add minced garlic and sauté for an additional 1-2 minutes until fragrant.

➤ Pour in vegetable broth, add white beans, chopped tomatoes, dried thyme, dried rosemary, bay leaf, salt, and pepper.

➤ Bring the soup to a boil, then decrease the heat to low, cover, and simmer for 15-20 minutes to allow the flavors to blend.

➤ Stir in chopped kale and continue to boil for an additional 5-7 minutes until the kale is soft.

➤ Discard the bay leaf.

➤ Taste and adjust the seasoning if needed. If you like, add a squeeze of fresh lemon juice for a flash of brightness.

- ➤ Ladle the White Bean and Kale Soup into bowls.

- ➤ Optional: Garnish with grated Parmesan cheese.

- ➤ Serve your cozy and healthful White Bean and Kale Soup hot.

- ➤ Enjoy this nourishing and comforting soup on a chilly day!

Sesame Ginger Tofu Stir-Fry

Ingredients:

For the Tofu:

- 1 block extra-firm tofu, pressed and cubed
- 2 tablespoons soy sauce (low-sodium)
- 1 tablespoon sesame oil
- 1 tablespoon cornstarch

For the Stir-Fry:

- 2 teaspoons vegetable oil
- 1 bell pepper, sliced
- 1 cup broccoli florets
- 1 carrot, julienned 3 green onions, sliced 2 tablespoons sesame seeds (for garnish)

For the Sauce:

- 2 tablespoons soy sauce (low-sodium)
- 1 tablespoon rice vinegar
- 1 tablespoon fresh ginger, minced
- 2 cloves garlic, minced
- 1 tablespoon honey or maple syrup
- 1 teaspoon cornstarch (optional, for thickening)

➢ **Instructions:**

➢ Press the tofu to remove excess water by laying it between paper towels and pressing a heavy object on top for at least 30 minutes.

➢ In a bowl, combine cubed tofu with soy sauce, sesame oil, and cornstarch. Gently toss to coat the tofu evenly. Let it marinade for 15-20 minutes.

➢ While the tofu is marinating, prepare the sauce by whisking together soy sauce, rice vinegar, minced ginger, minced garlic, and honey (or maple syrup). If you prefer a thicker sauce, you can add cornstarch.

➢ Heat vegetable oil in a wok or big skillet over medium-high heat.

➢ Add marinated tofu to the wok and cook for 5-7 minutes until golden brown on all sides. Remove tofu from the skillet and set it aside.

➢ In the same wok, add a touch more oil if needed. Stir-fry bell pepper, broccoli florets, julienned carrot, and sliced green onions for about 5-7 minutes or until the vegetables are crisp-tender.

➢ Add the cooked tofu back to the wok.

➢ Pour the prepared sauce over the tofu and vegetables. Toss everything together to coat evenly.

➢ Cook for a further 2-3 minutes until the sauce thickens slightly.

➢ Garnish the Sesame Ginger Tofu Stir-Fry with sesame seeds.

➢ Serve over brown rice or quinoa.

➢ Enjoy the bright flavors and textures of this wonderful tofu stir-fry!

Lemon Garlic Shrimp Skewers

Ingredients:

- 1 pound big shrimp, peeled and deveined
- 3 tablespoons olive oil 3 tablespoons fresh lemon juice
- 3 cloves garlic, minced
- 1 teaspoon lemon zest 1 teaspoon dried oregano
- 1 teaspoon smoked paprika
- Salt and pepper to taste
- Wooden or metal skewers

Instructions:

- ➢ If using wooden skewers, soak them in water for at least 30 minutes to prevent scorching.

- ➢ In a bowl, whisk together olive oil, fresh lemon juice, minced garlic, lemon zest, dried oregano, smoked paprika, salt, and pepper.

➤ Add the peeled and deveined shrimp to the marinade, ensuring each shrimp is completely coated. Let it marinade for at least 15-20 minutes.

➤ Preheat your grill or grill pan over medium-high heat.

➤ Thread the marinated shrimp onto skewers.

➤ Grill the shrimp skewers for 2-3 minutes per side or until they are opaque and have lovely grill marks.

➤ Optional: Squeeze additional fresh lemon juice over the skewers before serving for an extra punch of citrus flavor.

➤ Remove from the grill and let them rest for a few minutes.

➤ Serve your Lemon Garlic Shrimp Skewers with a side of quinoa or a fresh green salad.

➤ Enjoy these juicy and tasty shrimp skewers with the bright and acidic aromas of lemon and garlic!

Cauliflower and Broccoli Gratin

Ingredients:

- 1 head cauliflower, cut into florets
- 1 head broccoli, cut into florets
- 2 tablespoons butter
- 2 tablespoons all-purpose flour
- 2 cups milk
- 1 cup shredded cheddar cheese
- 1/2 cup grated Parmesan cheese
- 1 teaspoon Dijon mustard
- 1/2 teaspoon garlic powder
- Salt and pepper to taste
- 1/4 cup breadcrumbs (optional, for topping)
- Fresh parsley for garnish

Instructions:

➢ Preheat your oven to 375°F (190°C).

➢ Steam cauliflower and broccoli florets until they are slightly soft, around 5-7 minutes. Drain and set aside.

- In a saucepan, melt butter over medium heat.

- Stir add flour to produce a roux, and cook for 1-2 minutes until it turns golden brown.

- Gradually whisk in milk, ensuring there are no lumps. Cook, stirring regularly, until the mixture thickens.

- Reduce the heat to low and add shredded cheddar cheese, grated Parmesan, Dijon mustard, garlic powder, salt, and pepper. Stir until the cheese is melted and the sauce is smooth.

- In a large bowl, mix the steamed cauliflower and broccoli with the cheese sauce. Gently toss to coat evenly.

- Transfer the mixture to a baking dish.

- Optional: Sprinkle breadcrumbs over the top for a crispy topping.

➢ Bake in the preheated oven for 20-25 minutes or until the gratin is bubbling and golden brown on top.

➢ Remove from the oven and let it cool for a few minutes.

➢ Garnish with fresh parsley before serving.

➢ Serve your Cauliflower and Broccoli Gratin as a beautiful side dish or a warming main entrée.

➢ Enjoy the creamy and cheesy richness of this gratin!

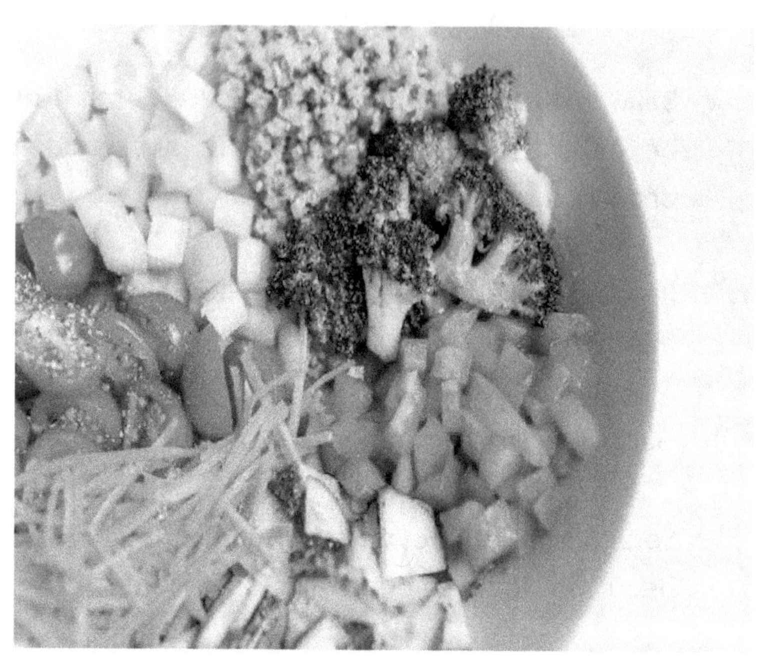

Chicken and Brown Rice Casserole

Ingredients:

- 1.5 pounds boneless, skinless chicken breasts, cooked and shredded
- 2 cups cooked brown rice
- 1 cup frozen peas
- 1 cup carrots, chopped
- 1 cup celery, chopped
- 1 onion, finely chopped
- 3 cloves garlic, minced
- 2 tablespoons olive oil
- 2 tablespoons all-purpose flour
- 2 cups chicken broth (low-sodium)
- 1 cup milk 1 teaspoon dried thyme
- 1 teaspoon dried sage
- Salt and pepper to taste
- 1 cup shredded cheddar cheese
- 1/2 cup breadcrumbs (optional, for topping)
- Fresh parsley for garnish

Instructions:

- ➢ Preheat your oven to 375°F (190°C).

- ➢ In a large skillet, heat olive oil over medium heat.

- ➢ Add chopped onion, diced carrots, and diced celery to the skillet. Sauté for 5-7 minutes until the vegetables are softened.

- ➢ Add minced garlic and simmer for an additional 1-2 minutes until fragrant.

- ➢ Stir in all-purpose flour to form a roux. Cook for 1-2 minutes until it turns golden brown.

- ➢ Gradually whisk in chicken broth and milk, ensuring there are no lumps. Cook, stirring regularly, until the mixture thickens.

- ➢ Season the sauce with dried thyme, dried sage, salt, and pepper.

- In a large bowl, combine shredded chicken, cooked brown rice, frozen peas, and the creamy sauce. Mix everything together.

- Transfer the mixture to a greased baking dish.

- Optional: Sprinkle breadcrumbs over the top for a crispy topping.

- Bake in the preheated oven for 25-30 minutes or until the casserole is bubbling and golden brown on top.

- Remove from the oven and let it cool for a few minutes.

- Sprinkle shredded cheddar cheese over the casserole and let it melt.

- Garnish with fresh parsley before serving.

- Serve your Chicken and Brown Rice Casserole as a healthful and comfortable supper.

- Enjoy the delightful blend of delicate chicken, brown rice, and tasty vegetables!

Sweet Potato and Black Bean Chili

Ingredients:

- 2 tablespoons olive oil
- 1 onion, chopped
- 3 cloves garlic, minced
- 1 big sweet potato, peeled and chopped
- 1 red bell pepper, chopped
- 1 green bell pepper, chopped
- 2 tablespoons ground cumin
- 1 teaspoon chili powder
- 1 teaspoon smoked paprika
- 1/2 teaspoon ground coriander
- 1 can (15 oz) black beans, drained and rinsed
- 1 can (14 oz) chopped tomatoes
- 3 cups vegetable broth (low-sodium)
- Salt and pepper to taste
- Fresh cilantro for garnish
- Avocado slices for topping (optional)
-

Instructions:

➢ In a big pot, heat olive oil over medium heat.

- ➤ Add chopped onion and minced garlic to the saucepan. Sauté for 5-7 minutes until the onion is transparent.

- ➤ Stir in ground cumin, chili powder, smoked paprika, and ground coriander. Cook for an additional 1-2 minutes to roast the spices.

- ➤ Add diced sweet potato, diced red bell pepper, and diced green bell pepper to the saucepan. Cook for 5 minutes, stirring periodically.

- ➤ Pour in vegetable broth, diced tomatoes, and drained black beans. Bring the chili to a boil.

- ➤ Reduce the heat to low, cover, and simmer for 20-25 minutes or until the sweet potatoes are cooked.

- ➤ Season with salt and pepper to taste.

- ➤ Ladle the Sweet Potato and Black Bean Chili into bowls.

➢ Garnish with fresh cilantro and top with avocado slices if preferred.

➢ Serve your tasty and nutritious chili with a side of whole grain rice or crusty bread.

➢ Enjoy the warmth and comfort of this Sweet Potato and Black Bean Chili on a chilly day!

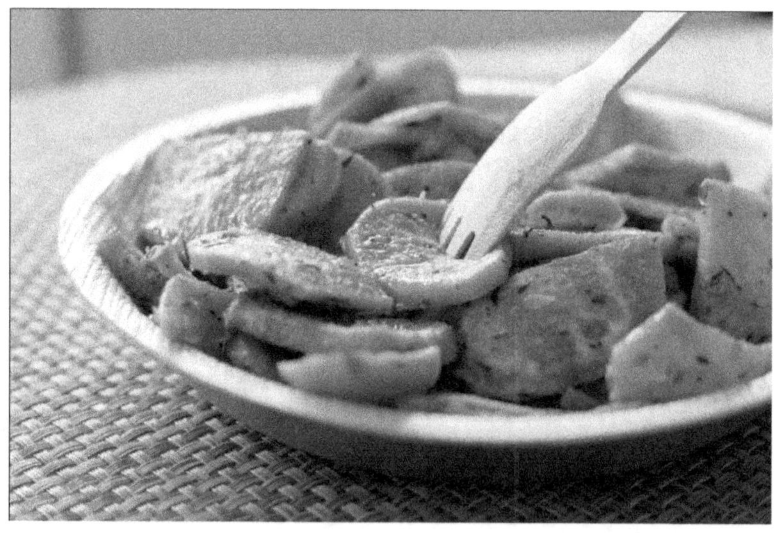

Grilled Vegetable and Quinoa Stuffed Bell Peppers

Ingredients:

- 4 big bell peppers, halves and seeds removed
- 1 cup quinoa, cooked according to package instructions
- 1 zucchini, diced
- 1 yellow squash, diced
- 1 cup cherry tomatoes, halved
- 1 red onion, chopped
- 2 tablespoons olive oil
- 2 cloves garlic, minced
- 1 teaspoon dried oregano
- 1 teaspoon dried basil
- Salt and pepper to taste
- 1 cup feta cheese, crumbled (optional, for topping)
- Fresh parsley for garnish

Instructions:

> Preheat your grill to medium-high heat.

- ➢ In a large bowl, combine diced zucchini, yellow squash, cherry tomatoes, and red onion with olive oil, minced garlic, dried oregano, dried basil, salt, and pepper.

- ➢ Grill the vegetables for 5-7 minutes or until they are slightly browned and tender. Remove from the grill and set aside.

- ➢ In the same bowl, mix the cooked quinoa with the grilled vegetables.

- ➢ Preheat your oven to 375°F (190°C).

- ➢ Place the bell pepper halves on a baking sheet.

- ➢ Stuff each pepper half with the quinoa and grilled veggie mixture.

- ➢ Optional: Top each filled pepper with crumbled feta cheese.

- ➢ Bake in the preheated oven for 20-25 minutes or until the peppers are cooked.

➢ Remove from the oven and sprinkle with fresh parsley.

➢ Serve your Grilled Vegetable and Quinoa Stuffed Bell Peppers as a healthful and colorful supper.

➢ Enjoy the bright tastes and textures of this delectable stuffed pepper meal!

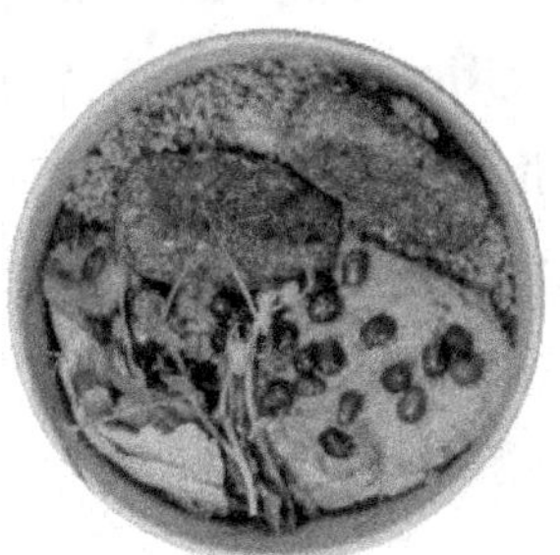 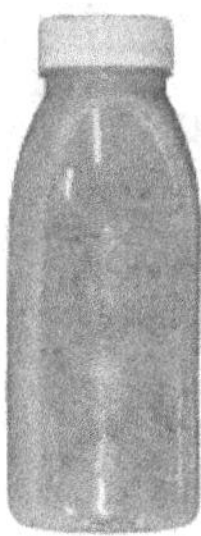

Tips for Dining Out:

It might be difficult to navigate restaurant menus while adhering to a renal-friendly diet, but you can make better judgments if you use these guidelines.

Look over menus online, select renal-friendly options, then make your order. For baked or grilled proteins, choose for lean meats, fish, and chicken, as these boost flavor without adding too much salt. To help you control how much salt you eat, ask for the sauce on the side. Customize your order by asking for lower-sodium options or specific cooking methods. Select fresh veggies for side dishes because they taste good even when they don't have a lot of salt. To curb intake and cut back on processed and canned foods, think about portion sizes.

Be wary of processed meats, high-sodium condiments, sodium that is concealed in seasonings, excessive dairy and cheese consumption, and rich, creamy foods if you want to avoid typical mistakes with the renal diet. When feasible, choose fried foods and broth-based options.

You may enjoy dining out and still eat a renal-friendly diet by being mindful of your environment and making informed choices. Share your dietary needs with the restaurant staff for a more tailored eating experience.

Hydration Tips:

Kidney health relies on maintaining adequate fluids. To stay hydrated, prioritize water, sip regularly, track urine color, avoid sugary drinks, choose low-phosphorus options, and opt for herbal teas. Kidney-friendly beverages include infused water, coconut water, cranberry juice, diluted lemonade, iced herbal teas, and sparkling water. Consult your healthcare provider for personalized fluid requirements.

Meal Prep Ideas:

Meal planning is crucial for maintaining a renal diet. To make it easier, create a weekly meal plan, cook in batches, pre-cut ingredients, freeze meals, and choose kidney-friendly staples. Use portion control containers for efficient nutrition intake management. Label containers with the dish's name and preparation date.

Consider one-pot meals for convenience and avoid unhealthy choices. Store kidney-friendly snacks in advance to avoid unhealthy choices. Experiment with different cooking techniques like slow cooking, pressure cooking, or rice cookers. Stay hydrated by including high-water content items in meals. Seek variety in meals to avoid boredom and maintain a healthy palate.

Consult a healthcare provider or dietician for personalized guidance based on your unique dietary needs.

Sarah's Path to Renal Health:

Introducing Sarah, a lively person residing in a busy metropolis. Sarah was told a few years ago that she had kidney problems and that in order to stay healthy, she needed to switch to a diet that was good for her kidneys. With a resolve to take charge of her health, she set out to adopt a lifestyle that was favorable to her kidneys.

A statement from Sarah

"I was feeling overwhelmed and apprehensive about what lay ahead when I initially found out about my renal condition. But I've seen amazing changes in my life because to the support of my medical team and a dedication to a renal diet.

Magic of Meal Preparation:

Meal preparation was one of the crucial elements that significantly changed the situation. I started organizing my weekly menu, emphasizing products that were low in phosphorus and fresh. My go-to tactic for conserving time and making sure I always had a kidney-friendly alternative available was batch cooking.

Tastes Without Giving Up:

The amount of taste I could still appreciate on a renal diet astounded me. I experimented with condiments, herbs, and spices to improve the flavor of my food without endangering the health of my kidneys. It added joy to every meal.

Making Empowering Decisions:

I got really good at reading restaurant menus and choosing options that wouldn't hurt my kidneys over time. I gained the ability to let waiters know about my dietary requirements so that I could have a fulfilling meal without risking my health.

Honoring Minor Victories:

Every improvement, no matter how tiny, was worth applauding. These tiny victories, like selecting a snack that wouldn't harm my kidneys or keeping up my hydration intake, gave me more strength to persevere.

a Community of Support:

Making connections with people who were on the same path as oneself proved to be motivating. By exchanging advice, recipes, and personal stories, a community of people who knew one another's struggles and successes was formed.

Living My Ideal Life:

I can now state with confidence that taking care of my kidneys is a way of life rather than a burden. Through prudent decision-making, an optimistic outlook, and continuous assistance, I have not only preserved my kidney health but also enhanced my general state of health. It demonstrates that anybody may successfully traverse the route to renal health with the correct resources and effort."

Sarah's success story demonstrates the life-changing potential of switching to a renal diet and adopting healthy lifestyle habits. Despite being fictitious, her tale captures the struggles and victories that many people actually encounter on their path to renal health.

Kidneys are vital organs responsible for regulating blood pressure, controlling electrolyte balance, and filtering waste. Common kidney disorders include chronic kidney disease (CKD), kidney stones, urinary tract infections (UTIs), and polycystic kidney disease (PKD). Maintaining kidney health involves a healthy diet, including controlled salt intake, phosphorus management, adequate fluid intake, protein moderation, potassium balance, monitoring blood sugar levels, and consuming good fats.

Reducing salt intake, choosing fresh, natural foods, limiting phosphorus intake, maintaining adequate fluid intake, consuming lean meats, poultry, fish, eggs, and potassium, monitoring blood sugar levels, and consuming good fats are essential for maintaining kidney health. Consultation with medical specialists is recommended for individualized guidance based on individual kidney disease and general health. This synopsis provides insight into the complex interactions between kidney health, common ailments, and diet, emphasizing the importance of ongoing discussions with healthcare teams.

The National Kidney Foundation, Mayo Clinic, AKF, MedlinePlus, NIDDK, and RSN provide resources on kidney health, treatment options, diet, diabetes, and renal support, while also emphasizing diet and diet control.

Good luck on your journey to Renal Health.

www.ingramcontent.com/pod-product-compliance
Lightning Source LLC
Chambersburg PA
CBHW070902260726
48661CB00004B/1560